SELF DEFENSE

The Art of Real Street Fighting Techniques

(The Ultimate Guide to Beginner Martial Arts Training Techniques)

Doris Amaya

Published by Tyson Maxwell

Doris Amaya

All Rights Reserved

Self Defense: The Art of Real Street Fighting Techniques (The Ultimate Guide to Beginner Martial Arts Training Techniques)

ISBN 978-1-77485-270-5

Legal & Disclaimer

medical advice before using any of the suggested remedies, techniques, or information in this book.

Upon using the information contained in this book, you agree to hold harmless the Author from and against any damages, costs, and expenses, including any legal fees potentially resulting from the application of any of the information provided by this guide. This disclaimer applies to any damages or injury caused by the use and application, whether directly or indirectly, of any advice or information presented, whether for breach of contract, tort, negligence, personal injury, criminal intent, or under any other cause of action.

You agree to accept all risks of using the information presented inside this book. You need to consult a professional medical practitioner in order to ensure you are both able and healthy enough to participate in this program.

TABLE OF CONTENTS

Introduction

The book is intended to aid the complete novice and those who have no training in combat. The book is intended as an introduction resource that will aid beginners in understanding pressure points and the best way to use the pressure points in self-defense situations.

You will be taught the definition of pressure points and how to utilize to protect yourself. Additionally, you will learn to effectively attack these points even with limited training. Also, you will learn how to aid a partner if you do knock him out in training.

Be aware that this isn't an exhaustive work, and you do not expect to know how to master the pressure points in this article without real practice and supervision by an instructor or mentor.

Thank you, and I hope you have fun with it!

Chapter 1: Gun Rights And The Us Constitution

The US Constitution, specifically the Second Amendment, gives its citizens the right to bear and keep arms. This is a debated right, and has been subject to debate for years.

One of the questions discussed in relation to this constitutional right is whether it is legally and legitimate to employ deadly force. In the words of US Armed Forces, deadly force is that is used by a person to cause grave bodily injury or death to someone else. Deadly force can also refer to situations where a prudent and reasonable person has reason to believe that there is a threat to cause grave physical harm and death.

There are a variety of opinions, rules as well as guidelines and rules regarding what constitutes a the use of force that is reasonable. The one thing that is common across all States is the the recourse to deadly force should only be used when it is a definite need, and as the last resort, and when the other options are proven to be ineffective or can't be used in a reasonable manner.

What qualifies as the most deadly force?

In essence, deadly force is the term used to describe weapons that may be used to cause death and/or severe bodily injury. They comprise explosives, firearms, vehicles as well as bladed weapons. Other items that aren't traditional and can be used to cause serious injury include everyday objects such as baseball bats tires, tire irons, and sharp pencils.

Critical questions

To be considered deadly force legitimate, it must include certain elements. These fundamental questions are essential to the different state laws across the US regardless of the different particulars and specifics in each state.

Did the decision to use force justified?

Was the use of lethal force really necessary?

Was the force that killed you reasonable?

Was the fatal accident or death likely to occur?

These questions form the basis that in every state, regardless of the laws are in place there are times when killing force cannot be regarded as an acceptable act for self-defense. For instance, the person who triggered an attack can't be excused from any legal liability if they employed violent force against someone else regardless of whether the other person attempted to kill, or at the most, inflict serious harm. Another condition is that the person who attacked be able to clearly state their intent and have the possibility of inflicting the death of a person or inflict serious injury. For instance, if someone had a gun, but wasn't pointing at anyone, then any person who shoots them can't use the legal recourse to deadly force. In addition, nobody is able to shoot someone that happens to be in the backyard without having a weapon or indication of malicious motive.

There are exceptions

There are situations where the use of force is not acceptable due to various specific reasons.

Law enforcement officers or police officers

It is extremely challenging to justify the usage of force against these individuals. They are mandated by law to ensure peace and peace and. They are also instructed to use the least amount of force in pursuing, apprehending, or capturing anyone. There are occasions when police officers might use excessive, or inappropriate force, the use of violent force against them is difficult to prove to be justified. There are a lot of instances where ordinary citizens complain of being subjected too much force from police when they confront their concerns. There are instances where people are subjected to unjustifiably excessive brutal force by law enforcers or police personnel. But, based on the state laws using violent force against them could likely result in being a crime unless there is a substantial and convincing evidence to support the use of force. One thing is certain anyone who used brutal violence against officers of the law or law enforcement officers when they were performing their duties in the course of their duties will likely be prosecuted.

The most important thing to consider determines the scope of job and the responsibilities they have. They are legally entitled to carry guns and make use of them when needed. While performing their legal responsibilities there will be times where they'd be pointing at other people, such as people who are not in the intention to cause injury. For the common citizen who is pointing guns could be seen as a threat to serious bodily harm , which could justify self-defense. But, the law views this as a stance of the police officer or law enforcement official as a part of their duty to perform and not as a sign of purpose of malicious intent. This is viewed by the law as an integral part of the police and law enforcement system.

To illustrate:

For example, a legal search was conducted on a residence, i.e., home. Police officers came into the house, guns drawn and prepared to shoot. Under normal circumstances, the homeowner has the right to defend his property using brutal force. However, since they were policemen, the homeowner will be required by law not to use the use of force against these individuals. They are performing their duty in accordance with their obligations and responsibilities imposed by law. If a homeowner shoots the officers even if they forcefully into his home at night, the homeowner cannot justify it as self-defense. night, the homeowner is not able to justify shooting them as self-defense.

The principle behind this is to stop civilian interference in the execution of law enforcement and police obligations. Imagine homeowners shooting officers who are crossing their lawns to catch a law offender, or suspect being taken into custody at his home, and then shooting the police officer, then getting away with the crime with the excuse of self-defense.

There are instances where the use of deadly force against police officers and law enforcement officers might be justifiable.

Bail bondmen

If these individuals are performing their jobs, any person who resorts to violence against them will not be able to justify self-defense to justify. Bail bond agents have the same fundamental protections and motives as law enforcement as well as police officials.

Landlords and other individuals who are also entitled to be there

Respecting the rights of other people also. For example landlords have the right to access the homes of his tenants to ensure safety, for instance. It's his right since even though someone is living or renting within the house, that property is still his property. He has the legal right, as per laws, to make it secure in the way he thinks best. The tenant also has the power to defend the property however should he be in conflict with the landlord, the majority of laws are against the landlord. For example, a landlord could infiltrate the tenant's home and the tenant can't block him from entering or even shoot him as a result of the landlord's presence.

Outside of these situations the use of deadly force in self-defense is not allowed by law if the perpetrator or attacker has already left or stopped the threat. For instance when a person points the gun at someone puts it down, or begins to flee then there is no legal reason to shoots him in a lethal manner. Refrain or a cessation of the threat behavior does not put the person in immediate risk.

Chapter 2: Beware

The first priority is to ensure that we are as informed as we can about all the possible ways that we could bring trouble into our lives. If you're well-armed with this information and are aware of the dangers, you'll be able to avoid engaging into any of these scenarios either unconsciously or in the past. In this article I've gathered some of the most groundbreaking research findings that I'd like for you to read not just to increase the awareness of you, but also also for decreasing your chance of becoming the victim of an act of crime or violence.

Do you think you're aware of the various types of events that could endanger your security? It is essential to be aware to detect the real threat. In the end, our actions and actions are crucial to the final outcome. Physically defending ourselves using the techniques we have learned is a last solution in every scenario.

How to Avoid Being an obvious target

You might be not aware of your own easy target?

Do you usually go out after dark? It's obvious however, dark corners of the streets aren't the most ideal locations. We all take our dogs out at night or make quick visits to the supermarket or gas station without thinking about it however it is best to not delay these chores until the time that the sun sets. Be out earlier , if you can, and then be back home by sunset.

Do you walk, walk, or exercise while playing music listening to music with headphones? A lack of focus or apathy can greatly increase your risk.

When you are considering moving to an area that you're considering It's not just a good idea to investigate the area on the internet It's important to drive around and talk to prospective residents about their experience in the neighborhood. Explore the neighborhood at night to see what the lighting in the area is, and which areas you might want to avoid at specific periods of time. Sometimes , you'll be surprised by at the information you gather that could influence your purchase decision.

Street corners and roads aren't all the places where that people are targeted. It can happen in workplaces, apartments, homes and even when visiting friends' homes as well.

We are often able to trust our friends, but at times, those closest to us could pose risky to your security. Be wary of the people you surround yourself with. This may sound weird or a bit skeptical however, sometimes , even psychopaths create a very cozy atmosphere build trust, and convince you that they are too good someone to pose an actual threat. Therefore, a large part of your personal security is making sure that you don't allow the wrong individuals into your personal circle from the start.

Believe in your intuition. If you're female, you're blessed with an incredible sense of smell that can help your life in the event of imminent danger. Your eyes are often able to detect odd behavior as well as body expressions that sends off warning signals through your body. Be aware of this and stay in a relationship with someone who triggers the alarm bells in your head, even in the case of a friend who you've been with for quite a while.

Criminals usually have no motive to commit an offence. A negative mental state or a tendency to have negative thoughts could cause them to become a criminal.

You may be shocked by how many people ignore their basic sense on a regular basis. If you're in a restaurant or bar and you're able to accept food or drinks from someone else could be very risky. If someone is showing an interest that is only yours do not be enticed to express gratitude for it. Instead, keep your eyebrow up. It is important to remain aware and be able to decline courteously, without provoking unnecessary tension. If there's someone you're attracted to, be patient until you've got to know this person over a long amount of time. Be confident. When you discover you're in a bad situation Be smart, take action. Choose a courteous way to remain "busy" or "unavailable" and eliminate the person as soon as you can.

If someone, whether male or female, starts to make you uneasy, even after having been out on a few dates, make sure to begin writing the dates and the unsettling behaviour down. Then, begin making a note of the incident. Also, you should inform anyone you trust right away. If the person you're talking to is found to be dangerous, you'll want someone else to be aware of what's going on with the person in order to give useful information to law enforcement officials and anyone else who is who are looking out for your best interests.

These preventative measures keep all your lives in the own hands.

Here's a neat chart of comparisons that shows the common sense kind of thought that helps keep your brain conscious. It's a brief review of examples that prevent you from reasoning.

Kh

Avoid using public restrooms during the night. Always ask a trusted friend to be waiting outside.

You are driving home late at night , you are by yourself unconsciously deciding for a short bathroom stop.

Avoiding high-crime or "bad" zones. Doing your best to get a refill at a gas station that is cheaper in a less shady area of town.

Saying no thanks to an appealing offer of food or drink from a nice stranger.

Then you are caught up in the moment and allowing your feelings of flattery allow you to accept drinks and food offered by strangers.

Be aware of your consumption of alcohol to prevent getting drunk from your home. Beware of drinking intoxicated at a gathering or out on an evening out with a friend.

Examining streets and roads in a new location before buying a home simply because it looks attractive.

Do not rely on a person's appearance and relying on your own instincts. Don't trust someone on their face and disregarding warning signals.

How to Identify a Suspicious Person

They show who they really are through their behaviour, their actions, and their words. However, someone with an aggressive personality may appear normal on the surface. People who do not really love you, or who are incredibly jealous of you, won't admit it in front of you.

Burglars and thieves attack you from the beginning. Someone who is trying to hurt you might appear to be someone you know initially, and keep their intentions secret. How do you identify who's trying to harm you?

Be aware that learning self-defense skills will make you the first line of defense. A vigilant and focused mind will help you to see the warning signs in a clear manner prior to the moment the fight takes off.

Someone who appears to be overly curious: You should be on guard if someone who you don't get to really know, seems to seem overly curious about you. If you've had a recent encounter with an individual in your office.

* Does he ask to many questions about his personal life?

* Does she appear overly excited about your background, family issues and so on. ?

* Do you think that he's trying to connect with you despite the fact that you don't like him?

If yes, you need to be on guard and vigilant. Take a notebook and take notes on exactly what took place and do your best to avoid attracting the person's focus.

An Individual with an aggressive nature: When it comes to the people you've already met there is a possibility that anyone could have an aggressive or latent nature that could be a warning sign for trouble.

Do they exhibit an polarizing personality?

Have you ever observed the person become aggressive in normal conversations?

Being around the same type of person can lead to assaults by well-known attackers against strangers. They may not have negative intentions towards you personally but their personality, or an uncontrollable attitude can cause the perfect storm that leads to a potentially dangerous attack.

It's true, it happens every day.

A person who is extremely Lovely: If a person who you don't know attempts to be so kind or helpful that you feel a surge of emotion It's best to keep away from them. This isn't the kind of person this time, but it's the intentions of the person you must be wary of. Don't share your personal details to anyone else regardless of how nice or harmless they encounter.

Be cautious not to become scared or overly suspicious. If someone seems to be genuinely friendly, there's nothing wrong with it. But, if the person displays too much interest or attempts to obtain information about your life, either in exchange for or as a result of, the favor they offered Be on guard and stay completely quiet, even if it's just an exchange that appears to be polite.

People who seem to be extremely jealous of Your Success or You It's true. The human nature of envy is part of our human nature. However, it's crucial to recognize that a desire for pleasure could turn into a powerful threat to people who cannot stop their jealousy.

Be aware of the tendency to be jealous by looking at a person's personality, body language, verbal expressions and responses.

* How can an acquaintance or a close family member react to your success?

*Some people may appear to be pleased for you however if they are jealous of your accomplishments, their behavior could differ from time to time. You can discern their true thoughts by observing their facial expressions as well as how they speak and, perhaps most important, their attitude toward you over the course of weeks, days, and hours that are following.

Be aware of the factors previously mentioned. For absolute security it is essential to recognize that anyone can become an enigma. They could be so close to you that your mind may be resistant to recognizing them as any risk to your security. Be prepared to conquer this resistance. This is why you need to be aware and be able to spot any indicators of danger that might be there.

The Most Common Kinds of Criminal Acts

It's true that this isn't an easy subject to discuss but we're talking about raising awareness in this case.

* Murder: Someone could or may not have a valid reason for murder, but murders are committed daily across the globe. A lot of victims miss warning signs that could have been a lifesaver.

*Rape: The majority of people are victimized through someone whom they are familiar with. What warning signs do they overlook? A better education and more judicious judgment can prevent many instances of sexual assault.

Acute Assault Strikes and fights break out all day each day, causing injuries to the body and. In-person confrontations with an aggressive or violent person typically result in this kind of scenario. Someone may be hostile towards you however, most of the time it's an uninvolved acquaintance, colleague, friend or family member with no control over their behavior and is the one to blame. It is for this reason that it is best to avoid interacting with these types of people.

• Robbery occurs either on the road and at your home. Through acquaintances (housekeepers or babysitters and so on.) or foes (complete strangers). We'll discuss more in depth the best ways to stop the possibility of robbery in the final chapter.

If you are faced with a situation that is difficult to ignore, it's best to

Don't overlook that it's important assess the severity of an issue early. To avoid causing unneeded conflict, it is important to be aware of when a response is required and when it isn't. There are always situations that you need to be tactful about dismissing. For instance?

* It is best to ignore cats calling. They're harmless and shouldn't be ignored. The smart aleck's comments that do not make any explicit attempt to get into your space or track your movements should be firmly disregarded. Don't let it trigger your attention. Avoid them and get yourself out from the surroundings if needed.

* A irritable or jealous person usually does not have a reason to harm you. If you observe indications that a colleague or friend is jealous of you or your life overall you should stay away from their company. Do not try to confront the person about the matter. It's completely unnecessary. You don't need to worry about them. It's just a matter of avoiding them.

* If your coworkers, friends, or family members seem to be unruly It is best to avoid them instead of being aggressive and create a negative impact on the

situation. Avoid being in the company of this person for as long as you can.

Situations that are extremely stressful are easily avoided by simply knowing when to move on and when to ignore annoying people.

What can increase the chance of Violence?

We've discussed how to stay away from becoming vulnerable to attack the common criminals that plague our society, the types of people whom you must be wary of, and the situations where it's acceptable to just ignore the irritations. We'll now look at factors that could significantly increase the likelihood of being a victim.

* Self-control. As we've stated, your safety is mostly in your hands. Do not lose your sense of logic and precise reasoning.

* Surrender. It's not a good idea to allow the opponent to see any sign of weakness in your character, even if you must create a strong cover to conceal it. If they can tell you're scared and they are, it can increase the confidence of those who succeed by sabotaging you.

* Do not become aggressive. This will increase the risk of violence. You must be sure but remain in a calm state. A calm mind thinks more clearly about the best way to get out of or avoid the dangers of a situation.

Avoid confrontations over words. It's crucial to choose your battles. It's sometimes tempting to defend yourself of someone else or yourself However any argument that is verbal with a jealous, angry or angry person is likely to cause more stress and worsen the situation.

Chapter 3: Self Defense Tips To Keep Yourself Safe On Streets

Self-defense is a vital capability, and nobody should doubt this. It is a fundamental right of every human being to protect oneself his home, property, and those he loves from threats to their lives. It is a sad situation in the world of today that we have people who engage in predatory behavior and are not hesitant about harming another human being.

People falsely believe that this kind of violence is not likely to occur to them. This is both reckless and foolish. It's reckless simply because you're not thinking in recognizing the real dangers that are out there. This kind of thinking is foolish since it scoffs at and even ignores the real threats that exist in the present day society.

It's a fact having a good understanding of self-defense can make your life or death, or the risk of tragedy and safety. Self-defense, as you might already know is not necessarily a requirement that you need to fight or take on the opponent. These are seven useful strategies (or you could call them guidelines if you like) to ensure your safety. These advices are from martial arts specialists who've been training street-smart self-defense for a long time.

Self Defense Tip #1 - Awareness of Surroundings-Preventing Imminent Threats

Everybody has heard the phrase"prevention" is the best alternative to finding an answer. This is the same in the realm of self-defense as well as the martial arts. The best fighter is the one who is able to avoid a fight.

It doesn't matter if either on your own or in a group, the most important aspect is to detect any danger and take action prior to the threat becomes imminent. If your gut instincts suggest that someone in the alley behind you is suspect, then it's important to take note of it.

The ability to sense your own instincts is an essential piece of self-defense. But that does not mean that you must be at a point of apprehension and be suspicious of every thing you notice. It's enough to establish a routine to observe the surroundings in the surrounding area, including things that are located a long distance away.

When driving, you typically focus your attention on the road, and this happens naturally. Keep your eyes at the vehicle in front of you, but you also take the time to be aware of other vehicles and objects which are further away. This is a skill that can be learned however, it keeps you secure in the roadway.

It is possible to apply the same concept everywhere you travel. It is a good habit to be aware of all around you. It's only one quick glance. Look for potential dangers close to you as well as those that are far away. If you spot a potential danger, determine how you will respond. This can also stop anyone from catching you off guard.

Tips for Self-Defense #2 - Walk in Confidence, but beware of eye Contact

If you've spotted the signs of danger, or are in an uninviting part of the area, be sure to move with confidence. If you are scared but you are able to pretend to be confident. All you need to do is look confident. Keep your head straight and your chest up. Maintain your posture and keep your chin straight.

Be aware that the majority of attackers will just target those they believe are weak and unprotected. Sure, you could label them cowards, but that's exactly the way they see it. Predators don't want to spend their time and energy for someone who could be an issue. They simply want things accomplished quickly and with minimal fuss. If you seem to be someone who is able to put up some serious resistance, they'll most likely abandon you and look for another possible target.

But, being confident isn't enough. It's important to remain conscious of what's going around you (see the tip 1 . above). If you encounter people who are still trying to talk with you despite of appearing like someone who doesn't mind being bullied It's time to take a stand to avoid any confrontation (see #3 below). Be confident and appear like someone who is able to stand up to a significant amount in resistance are another tool for self-defense you can utilize.

Self Security Tip #3 - Beware of Confrontation as Much as you can

Kenny Rogers once wrote a song titled "Coward of County." The song is about one man who was branded by everyone in the neighborhood as a "coward" who was never a confrontation with anyone, let alone engaged in any one who tried to intimidate him. It appears that he did not take on the bullies due to the promise he made to his father. One of the lyrics of this song is about the advice that the man's father gave his son and that is to avoid trouble whenever you want to, but it does not mean that you're weak, it's just that you don't need to engage in an effort to prove your worth.

It's the same in self-defense. Avoiding confrontations is a way to defend yourself! It is important to note that half of people who go into combat will eventually are beaten up or worse, regardless of abilities or backgrounds. Even a professional in combat arts has an equal chance of standing in a fight. Everyone is equal in the fight.

If you aren't happy with those odds , you should avoid any confrontation. Chances of walking free of injury are greater if you stay clear of the possibility of a confrontation. If you're being accosted by an assailant , the very first step is to negotiate your way to get out of the way. If the person who is threatening you wants your money, then you should give it up. your wallet. Keep in mind that your alternatives are your wallet, and your lifestyle.

Make every effort to avoid any physical fight. Get away, seek assistance, try to talk with the person who attacked you, apologize for the offender (in case it's because of you) and scream when you must and draw attention to the others who are around you. If you find yourself in a potentially dangerous situation, your self-esteem should not be the first thing you think of. Be aware that all self-defense experts suggest that fighting, and all forms of physical fights should be your last option.

Tips for Self-Defense #4 Strike First Ask Questions Later

If you find yourself in a situation where you're being snatched by someone nearby to help the attacker who is threatening you, they cannot be argued with or there's no way to escape, it's time to fight. Remember this rule: when you are forced to fight, you're not expected to fight in order to prove that you're the superior fighter. Take on the role of the pirates in the Pirates of the Caribbean movie fight to ensure that they are able to escape.

It is the norm that you must take a stand to defend your physical self be the first to take on. In a game of chess the player who is the first to move (the player with white pieces) enjoys a technological advantage over the other player. He has momentum , and the initiative of the other player is a massive decision in your favor. If you've exhausted all options , you are negotiating to get to a resolution, strike!

Self Defense Tip #5 - Attack with all Your Might

If you are going to attack, be sure you put everything in the trash. Put everything -

even the kitchen sink and infant in bathwater (well in a literal sense obviously). Be aware of what's at stake: your life. That means you need to be able to fight with conviction and with the intent to hurt the opponent. In any fight, those who don't have determination to win ends being thrown to the ground and being thrown out of the way, or even worse even dead. You or he will be the victim So give it everything you have.

The other thing you must keep in mind is that you should not attack your attacker only once. You must hit repeatedly in a row as possible. Choose your target, then attack the target with all of your strength and strike it repeatedly. Continue hitting that region of your opponent's body until is completely immobilized. It could take as many as five full power strikes for that.

TIP 6 for self-defense – Make sure you hit something that is important.

You shouldn't just hit anyone or anything. Some people believe that hitting someone's face is the ideal way to do it. It's fine - it's the best method for breaking your hands. We'll discuss the best way to punch with a fist, and other techniques in the near future. In the meantime, be aware that the face isn't the best area to attack.

Combat experts recognize that there are some parts of our bodies that are vital for putting your opponent to death as fast as you can. They refer to these areas of the human body the strike zones of critical importance, which comprise the groin, throat as well as the eye. If you strike these areas repeatedly with full force, they will be unable to move your opponent regardless of how massive or powerful they appear.

7 Self-Defense Tips Ask for help or get away

After you've got your opponent lying on the ground, do not wait around to see what else they could do. Do not even attempt to be the hero and capture the criminal. It is likely that your attacker is surrounded by friends that could be around. It's not a good idea to contend with more adversaries all in one day. One attacker is already one of many!

Chapter 4: The Basic Defensive Measures

We have been blessed with an organ that is capable of protecting itself. Forearms can serve as shields well cushioned and able to deflect blows. Also, our hands are able to curl inwards to create blunt sides when we form the fist, in order to strike those punches when needed. The body is prepared to perform any action you just need to learn how to utilize it correctly.

Here you can find an overview of of the most fundamental defense measures.

Make use of your arms as shields

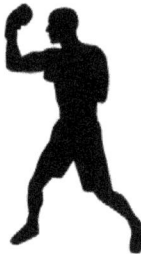

As we mentioned at the start in this section, the arm has been specifically designed to deflect the impact of punches. The forearm is composed of muscle, fat, and bone, all tightly wound together, when extended in the right time, can make punches look off. If you're good at recognizing and are skilled, it's relatively simple to utilize your arms as a protection against attack.

To block an attack, swiftly lift your broad side of your forearm the direction you want it to go and allow it to join with the punch coming from the opposite direction This will allow the attacker's hand to fly off harmlessly towards the side. It's crucial to time your timing to ensure that your forearm is positioned to the attacker's fist just below it.

If the attacker hits directly into your forearm it could result in painful. And if the strike is sufficiently powerful the arm could be broken. Much like everything else, it's dependent on timing. Once you've seen the fist flying towards your face from the corners of your eyes then raise your arm and let it block the punch, bringing it to the fist that is coming towards you. Arms can be very effective shields in the right way if you utilize them correctly. This is a crucial technique for self defense.

Dodge, Twist, Duck and Evade

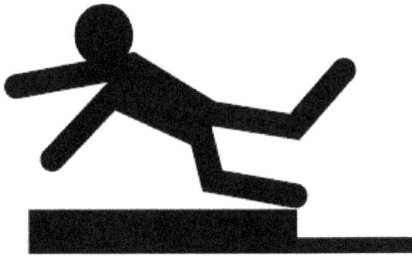

If you're unable to stop any punches that are thrown at you If you're unable to block punches, you may want to do all you can to avoid twist, dodge and avoid the attackers. It is all about the ability to think quickly. When you spot that strike coming towards you and you turn your body every direction possible, so as to stop the attacker from hitting.

They can be effective to avoid being struck, but the issue is that continuously dancing like a boxer in a arena can be quite exhausting. However it is possible to are able to maintain the endurance and strength to maintain a routine, you might exhaust your opponent enough that he may quit the fight entirely.

This was evidently the case for American fighter Muhammad Ali. At his peak, Ali would literally run around his bigger and stronger opponents. He was adept at evading, ducking and getting himself out of opponent's way. They could not lay a hand on him. In the in the meantime, they'd become so exhausted and exhausted that they would be close to collapsing.

As Ali aged his strategy started to be ineffective and he could not keep up with his high energy actions for long. If you're not an energy-hungry mush as Ali was in the early times of boxing it's likely that you won't be able to sustain this defense strategy for too long. You must use your own judgment to determine whether or not you need to utilize this strategy.

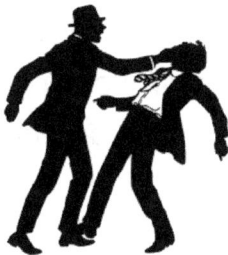

Learn to Grapple

The art of wrestling isn't only reserved for the WWF since being able to the hold of, handle and fight with a foe can be a game changer. For as crucial as the ability to block and avoid punches might be, it's not something that we can practice for a long time.

As such, performing our most authentic appearance as Muhammad Ali, ducking and trying to dodge bows from your opponent might not be the most effective strategy. Instead of doingdging or blocking it is better to grasp your opponent's arms and then bend them behind like a pretzel you'd be finished in a short time.

Many people believe that to accomplish this feat requires tremendous muscular strength. Although there's some factual basis to this, it's not the complete truth. You do require the strength of your arms in order to be able grapple but there's much more than this. The primary factor you'll have to improve does not have to be your strength in the biceps but it's your determination to be successful.

You can tell yourself that have control over the situation when you take hold of your opponent. Soon enough, you'll be. You have to channel your adrenaline and your anger over being attacked and apply it to your adversaries. If old women suddenly have sufficient blood-pumping power to take cars off of people in a crisis and you are capable of getting more than adequate blood circulation to wrestle against any potential attacker!

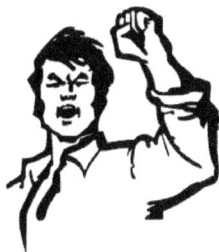

Use your hands to punch

The best defense is a solid offense. This could be the case in incidents of random attacks. Think about it this way, an attacker throws a punch at you and then expects you to be on defense.

What if you changed the script so that instead of backing off you accelerated forward and began taking the crap out them instead? It's sure to cause the victim with a shock and one that they're most likely not be in a position to recover. This method could work in the event that the attacker is able to get the knock on you and is able to hit you with a punch.

Didn't you manage to block or duck at the right time? Do not fret about it! Instead, just start pounding your opponent to oblivion. He's not likely to engage in a fight for long if it's the only thing he has to accomplish to prevent your jaw from breaking.

According to the current situation one of the most efficient methods to stop the attackers is launch a more aggressive and overwhelming assault. A stance like this will cause the attacker to be more aware of what they're doing. In the back of their mind, the attacker knows they're not doing the right thing and, when confronted with an imposing opponent the attacker will rapidly cease to bother you further.

Chapter 5: Vulnerable Point Self-Defense

Also called pressure points, these vulnerable areas of the body can be beneficial for self-defense particularly if the person you are fighting is much bigger or athletic than you. In addition, they can be utilized to keep attackers from being caught off guard because the degree of pain they cause is usually much more than the pain they cause in the event of striking them in a normally weak area.

Head

Forehead: Using the center of the forehead can cause the head to move backwards without much resistance, as long as the attacker isn't anticipating it. If done with sufficient force, it may cause the brain to move inside the skull, causing an injury or disorientation. The most efficient method to strike the forehead is with the palm's heel. Alternately you can hit the inside of the skull in the middle for the similar impact. You'll want to avoid the ridges at the front of the skull, or the area directly over the forehead, as they're strong enough to stop this strike from taking effect.

Temples found on both sides of the head, near at the tops of ears, are the points at which the cranium becomes the most thin and most fragile. Therefore, a carefully placed hit using an ear knuckle could cause brain hemorrhage, concussion or even death, if executed in a way that is sufficient. When practicing this technique, it is crucial to avoid contacting the sparring partners. It can be difficult to hit if you do not have enough practice , so it is suggested to stay clear of it during fights until you're certain you are able to hit it correctly.

Alternately, you could render your opponent unconscious by delivering an exact blow to the temple , which is called a phoenix eye punch. The punch is made by stretching the knuckle of your fingertip until the point forms kind of point. The move is also recognized to cause death, which is why it is imperative to only do it when you are certain that your life is in danger.

Neck

Although any neck blow is effective if done with sufficient force, to really incapacitate your attacker, the best option is to employ what's called a sleeper hold. For this technique you will need to put yourself in front of your adversary and put your arm in a wrap around the neck of their attacker. Once you are in position you're likely to make use of the forearm's bone also known as the radius to exert pressure on their carotid artery externally. The artery can be felt in the back of the throat, where you will feel the beat of the pulse. It is possible to increase the pressure upon the arterial by bringing your arm rapidly towards your body and grasping the wrist of your dominant hand with the other hand. Breathing into and out of your breath can also increase pressure. You might also wish to put your dominant hand inside the elbow of the other arm to secure your neck more securely.

If you are stuck in a sleeper-like position You can fight it with a turn of your head toward the elbow, which cuts off blood flow. The resultant space will prevent the hold from working properly and will also give you breathing space. It will not eliminate the pressure in the artery completely however, the time is still important. You will then want to grasp the elbow which is surrounding your neck by using the hand closest to it. After that, it uses any of the pressure points in the neck, which will be discussed further in the chapter. This will loosen the grip somewhat , allowing you to then follow it up with a blow on the groin or by stepping on their feet to break up the hold completely.

Another method to strike the neck is using the flat part of your palm, with your pinky facing downwards for striking between your collarbone and the jar. This method is superior to hitting the neck directly, as it requires a higher level of precision than most people are able to do in a real fight. Based on your general strength level and the size of the opponent's neck, you might be able grasp and squeeze to end their air supply or grasp and pull with a lot of force to break it completely. Dislocating the neck can be fatal, however, caution is highly recommended in the majority of cases.

Shoulder

Although not technically the shoulder the move could cause severe pain for people who are unaware, usually enough to end an argument before it starts. In this situation you'll be looking for the collar bone, then insert your fingers into the space behind it and then pushing it downwards using all the strength you can. It is likely to take a lot of practice to get the proper posture, since you'll have to be exact the first time you expect this maneuver to work during a confrontation.

Jaw

Underneath the jawline: To be able to effectively attack your jaw, you should extend your arms forward and grab the neck of your attacker directly below the jawline. Then squeeze it and pressing upwards while pressing upwards. It's not just painful, but it could cause airway obstruction in the event that your fingers are strong enough to completely disable the attacker.

The temporomandibular joints: In order to perform this maneuver, you'll need to keep your head supported with your second hand, and at the same time employing your first hand for follow the length of the jawline until it reaches the point close to your ear. By pushing forward and into the ear can result in significant discomfort and make it difficult for the attacker to talk freely. The typical reaction in this situation is to push backward, this is the reason it is essential to start by putting your head in a secure grip.

Alternately, you could hit the temporomandibular joints directly by using your primary knuckle. Ideally, it's the second knuckle on your middle finger. Making this move and then connecting, you will most likely result in the displacement in the jaw. The attack of both sides of the head may be equally effective, so striking the side that feels the most natural to your dominant hand is suggested.

Forearm

The space that makes up the natural crevice in the forearm (directly from that of the elbow) is composed entirely of muscles and tendons which give you plenty of material with which to work. For best outcomes, you're going to want to hold your elbow in such so that the thumb of your hand is in the crevice. When you are aligned, you're likely to be pushing downwards using your thumb before pushing upwards with the other fingers. It is vital to increase the thumb's grip with the fingers that are ancillary to ensure that you have enough leverage to succeed.

Alternately , you can press your thumb in the exact center of the crevice in one or the other side of the crevice, and into the suction called the brachioradialis of the outside forearm that is apparent when you (like your opponent) strikes an attack with a fist. This is a difficult move to master when you are in the middle of an attack, and it is suggested that you test it out before you apply it in a fight.

Hands

Hand's backside The hand's back into the bone using either one knuckle strike using the second one with extended knuckles, or by a punch that is simple can be a fantastic way to force your attacker to let go when they are in a grip of you in a threatening manner. Although it could harm your opponent in the event that it hits in a safe manner, the pain is quickly gone making it a breeze to master in relative security.

Fingers are a good place to catch an attacker's' blows from mid-air, then the first thing you'll need to do is try wrapping both your hands around the object before lifting it in your armpit, and then squeeze it to hold it in place. It is then important to grasp the elbow joint between its top and inner points and then squeeze down with all the force you can on either side. If done correctly, this could cause enough pain to make it feel like that the elbow is breaking but that isn't actually happening.

Torso

Sternum: Making a single knuckle strike that hits your opponent's sternum could lead to the bone fracture because it's not protected by muscle or fat. This could result in serious internal injuries, so is only recommended when you believe your life is in peril.

Solar Plexus: The solar is the nerve bundle that lie deep in the abdomen. They are often thought to be the place where deep emotions originate. The solar plexus is a bundle of nerves below the sternum and where the ribs join to the front in the abdominal cavity. When you strike this region with a strong strike, you may cause the diaphragm muscle to contract violently that is similar to blowing the wind out of the body of someone. If you're aiming for the solar plexus, then you need to strike it fast because this action is countered by engaging abdominal muscles.

Chapter 6: Martial Arts Basics

Synopsis

If someone decides to improve their ability to defend themselves, master self-defense or to become a better person, one thing is likely to come to mind: martial art. Martial arts are very popular nowadays, and are used all over the world.

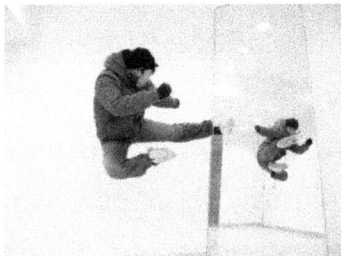

Martial Arts

Martial arts were practiced throughout the ages, but they really became popular during the period that of Bruce Lee. Bruce developed the method that is known as Jeet Kune Do, which is characterized by extremely fast strikes and amazing counter-defenses. When people began to realize the speed at which Bruce Lee may move, they began to research martial arts and see what benefits it could bring to them.

Martial arts can be broken down into distinct styles. The form of training you select is contingent upon the location and the subject you are studying. Many nations and cultures offer martial arts which they developed or developed and refined. Brazil provides Brazilian Jui-Jitsu, Japan has Karate, Thailand has Muay Thai, France has Savate and China includes Shaolin. Keep in mind that every style differs in the way it is taught and what it can provide you.

Although many people view martial arts as merely to protect themselves, it isn't the whole truth. Martial arts are used in tournaments and competitions as well that may involve floor routines, sparring as well as block and brick breaking demonstrations. Around the world there are competitions and chances for champions demonstrate their skills and knowledge.

All martial arts can teach you to defend yourself, and importantly, they will help you develop self-control. When you begin to learn an art of combat it will quickly help you achieve a more positive mental state. Whatever type of martial art that you learn instructors will teach self-control into your mind.

For those who are prone to an issue with tempers or require self-control martial arts could be a great way to learn. While you'll learn self-control, you'll also be able you can defend yourself even in most difficult of scenarios. Self-control is essential because martial arts can be deadly if handed out to the wrong person and with the wrong intent.

In the past decade there has been numerous mainstream competitions which showcase martial arts, such as Extreme Fighting, King of the cage and, the most viewed of them all that of course, the UFC (Ultimate Fighting Championship). The UFC has been advancing through the years, drawing excitement from across the world. It brings stylists from around the world, to test their abilities and determine who's the superior fighter.

With the UFC many people have gotten an incorrect view of martial arts. A martial art is beneficial to master, however when it is used in the UFC however, it does not necessarily mean it's going to protect your life in the street. Karate for example, teaches striking and blocking with a minimal emphasis on grappling techniques. If you're close to your opponent, Karate truly doesn't help. At a certain distance, nevertheless, Karate may be really destructive.

Whatever way you view it, martial arts can be beneficial in the event that you study it with the proper motivations. Each style differs in its approach and what it will offer and that's why it is important to choose the most appropriate style to suit your needs and goals. want to accomplish. Martial arts can teach you the basics of self-defense and your self-defense. All you need to try is give it a test.

Chapter 7: Tips to Prevent The Rapp

The increase in rape cases which is often the result of the clothes worn by the women were wearing were extremely thin and unprotected. The customs and culture of a nation also affect. However, this is not a problem in the event that the person doesn't have a snobby appetite.

The main point is that whichever the motives behind the instances of rape, it would be more beneficial if both parties men and women to one another to remind your promise to not do anything that violate moral and religious values. The possibility of rape is for anyone, anyplace, and at any time when there's an opportunity, so you should not allow them to have a shot. So here's how you can avoid the possibility of rape:

1. Environmental alert

Women should be aware of the route and where to road when she is leaving. What you should known are crucial places such as police stations gas stations, supermarkets, public telephones and many more. This is in case you require assistance immediately. A way to maintain vigilance isn't difficult to be able to establish at a public location, however, do not appear arrogant or excessive. Don't be apprehensive about accepting assistance (food and drink offerings delivery, food and beverage offering, etc.) who are not aware as we do not know the origins and motives are hidden from the person.

2. Pick a spot that is packed.

Don't get used to wandering through the deserted locations like the shortcuts within the empty garden, a quick cut through the middle of rice fields, the narrow cut in front of an empty home, or the high-walled avenues. It could be risky in the event that there are individuals with a motive to commit crimes due to the fact that the victim is having difficulty finding assistance.

3. Looking for attention.

If the perpetrators are responsible for the offense, the victim needs to be alerted immediately for assistance. For instance, screaming for assistance! Thieves! Fire! Continue shouting until help arrives.

4. Take on the physical.

If the perpetrator has successfully held by the victim's body, they must will not give up with their body, squeezing and screaming, kick and striking or pinching, biting and scratching, pulling hair and other.

5. Keep your distance.

How to move left and right quickly in trying to maintain an adequate distance from the offender and the victim. The areas which must be guarded not to touch are between the chest and waist, where the victim's chest is the first area that the perpetrator touched it, he can easily control the victim.

6. Inflict pressure on weak areas of the of the offender.

Everybody has weaknesses when it comes to the eyelids and throat, as well as the solar plexus the ribs, and pubic victims. It is important to target the weak spots to ensure that the percentage of the perpetrators is will be split.

7. Utilize psychic powers.

The victim attempted to negotiate with the offender as the man was intelligent and thought, however, we are able to take advantage of the circumstance by using negotiations to the person who committed the offense. This procedure is a tiered process that ranges from mild warning to severe.

For instance, you could say "what is your reaction if your mother or your sister were sexually assaulted? What would you feel? or the expression "you were created in the female womb! !" or "I am an aids to patients! !" Or "I want to use condoms, but only if you first take a condom!" Remember this is the only way to get time and effort to get out of. If the perpetrator is off guard, immediately we could escape, we should.

8. Monkey theory.

In desperate situations and to fight for their lives when they are in danger, the monkey throws all of his possessions at anyone who does harm to him. Victims could be hit with objects that are positioned around them. This will reduce the number of perpetrators because the person who is responsible can shield the body from the objects.

If the victim must be cautious and fight for as long as they can however rape does still happen take your time and be patient. This is a test for God. Believe that God will test His people according to the capabilities of the servant itself. When you are closer to God following the incident, you've completed the test.

A traumatic incident that has caused physical and mental trauma. The victim may suffer from depression, anxiety, or may even be tempted to take their own life. However, I can assure you that when we awoke and ready to go on we felt the joy of God that we felt. Let the world know that we are able to get back up after falling, become an example for other women such as Oprah Winfrey, who has suffered the rape of her cousin and her fellow classmates at nine years old. young, yet she is not wallowing in her destiny, rather he did not give up and is now one of the most well-known and most wealthy women on the planet.

Chapter 8: The Common Goals

There are lots of various targets to study when studying pressure point self-defense. Every martial art has one form of pressure point combat. There is pressure point fighting in Karate They have it in Taekwondo and of course, Aikido instructors also make use of pressure points. Kung fu fighters utilize pressure points.

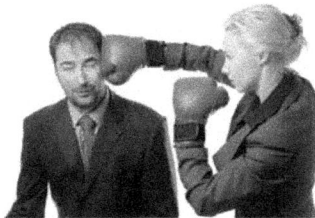

The most common targets to target in combat of this type are the painful points of the body. These include the temple as well as the ears, eyes as well as the throat, back of neck the chin and the nose.

These areas of the body are filled with nerve endings and pressure points. Injure any of these areas and you'll be severely injured. It is no surprise that certain points such as the eyes and nose, are quite delicate. If you hit them, it could result in serious injuries.

There's an additional element of the equation you must be aware of each target in self-defense based on pressure points is actually dependent on acupressure point. These are the same locations on your body where the acupuncturist will poke the body with needles.

Some pressure points have more pain than other points. Certain pressure points, when hit with enough force, could result in serious injuries and even death. Therefore, be cautious in your practice of the

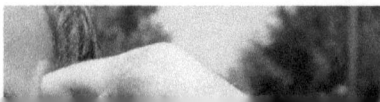

techniques that target those pressure points.

Be aware that the goal should not be to murder another person. It is your goal to defend yourself in order you are able to escape your life and bodily injuries diminished to zero or near to nothing.

Basic Strikes

We'll instruct you on two or three special strikes you can employ to target pressure points. But, you must be able to utilize the most basic strikes. This means that you must at a minimum know how to kick and punch.

In addition to kicks and punches the most basic strikes comprise elbows and knees. Sometimes, you'll need to also use headbutts if you are aiming at the face of your opponent.

If you decide to throw an attack or kick (or an elbow knee) make sure you use the correct technique. This means that you have to apply the entire weight of your body into the action and not rely solely on the strength of your leg or arm.

Striking with Intent

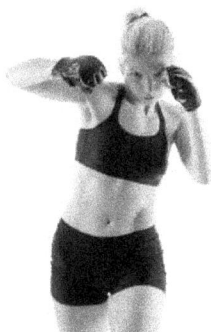

It is also important to move your body with a torque towards the direction of the strike. For example, if you're throwing a straight strike then you must lean forward and then apply the weight of your body when the fist hits the goal.

If you make straight punches with your right hand it means you need to keep your left foot in front with your right hand pulled inward in order to begin with. Then, raise your arm and then thrust your right hand into an open fist.

The majority of fighters will advise that you must be moving your fist. It is important to begin with a position in which you're right-handed palm is facing towards you. Then you'll turn it by using your thumb moving toward your floor (sort like a counterclockwise direction).

When you throw your right hand, you'll turn to the left foot (or your left foot when throwing your left hand - that is, you must turn your back leg). If when you make a hand-to-hand strike you should also turn your rear foot. Do not attempt to strike with a weak hand to hit anyone - remember that you're protecting yourself and your life is at stake.

While you kick, make use of the broad side of your foot, not your toes. Through some practice, you can also strengthen your shins, Yes it's true that you kick with them as well, since it's all bone. Of course , there are many ways to kick when practicing martial arts. Some kicks require you make use of the foot's ball or the edge of the sole, your shins and various other areas.

We won't go into too much specifics about this. We'll only provide instructions on the basic steps to execute simple kicks, so you'll be able to hit the necessary pressure points. This book doesn't focus on the kicks such as Muay Thai or Taekwondo.

Another thing to remember is that whenever you kick, be sure to move your leg as quickly as you are able to so your opponent won't have the chance to catch your leg while it's in mid-air.

Head

The head is among the main targets. There are several pressure points in the neck and the head. We'll discuss that in the future. In the meantime, it is important to be aware that the temple area is among the targets to be aiming for when trying to knock your opponent's head.

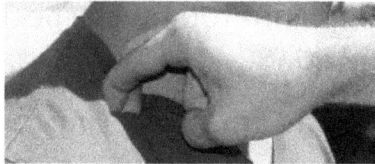

This is the face of the head. It's the opposite side of your opponent's forehead to be precise. It's actually one of the most thin parts of your skull. It may result in temporary dizziness. Some individuals may suggest making a fist using the middle finger extended in this manner:

Do not do it in a fight. If you do, you could break the bone on the fingers.

If you want to strike your opponent's temples, it is advised to make use of a hook. Make sure to strike that area using the actual knuckles on your hand. Hooks actually draw their strength from the swinging motion of your hand and the torque generated by your body's muscles as you move your torso and hips.

If it is executed correctly, your hook will appear like this:

If you can raise your fist sufficiently, you will be able to strike the temples of your opponent. By making a slight adjustments to the height, you can utilize the same hook to knock your opponent's jaw , causing the head to rotate. The jaw, naturally is a prime area of attack.

Necks are also popular target. In reality, as you'll discover in the following paragraphs, there are numerous pressure points along the neck you can strike to take out your opponent. You can train hitting the sides and back of the neck of your opponent. It is also advisable to try throwing punches at the neck of your opponent.

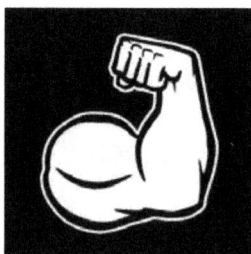

You can also take the neck of your opponent. You've seen these sleeper holds in professional wrestling shows, haven't you? You don't need to showmanship in it, but you could apply an open choke at the rear and force your opponent to fall out.

Shoulders

The next place to look at is something you're familiar with and can be extremely painful if you push down on it. Find your partner's collar bone. Then, you can poke downwards towards the side part of the bone using several fingers. It will be painful, but you must be close to your sparring partner or opponent. It is also important to be in a straight line with him in order to strike this area of your body.

Hands and Arms

The entire length of your arm is filled with Acupressure points and pain centers that you can make use of for your benefit. A large number of martial arts include techniques that make use of control of pain areas.

For example, Aikido practitioners and Brazilian Jiujitsu practitioners will employ techniques that stretch the wrists and elbows to angles which cause lots of discomfort, causing the opponent to accept or give up.

The insides of the crevice on the forearm that is opposite to your elbow (that portion in which your arm bends) is comprised of muscles and tendons which cannot be fully flexed. It's among the best spots to grab the arm and get the grip.

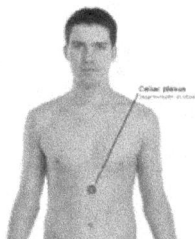

Celiac plexus

You can grasp that portion of your arm using all your fingers, except for the thumb at the elbow. The thumb stays in the crevices of the forearm or elbow. It is possible to hold the portion of your arm in this in the following manner:

It is essential to restrain or grasp the arm using your other hand in order that you are able to secure the hold. Another method to get to that point is to hit the area with your fist but your opponent must be in that the arm extends out and exposes the point.

But don't fret it's not the only crucial spot on the arm you could target. The internals of the biceps is an additional area that you could concentrate on. When your adversary is swinging violently then you can protect your head using your forearms. When you are at the right moment it is important to get used to timing this move and then raise your elbow, then step into the punch, and then aim your elbow toward the inner bicep of his, just like this:

It doesn't need to be exact. An elbow that is directly positioned to the bicep, even in the absence of flex is quite painful - so much that it could disable a person for a short time, writhing in pain. That should give you a chance to get out. Remember that the aim of self-defense isn't to to attack the person in front of you. Your main goal is to protect your personal safety and to get yourself out of the risky situation.

We'll discuss the techniques for tackling the insides of the biceps later, when we'll cover the exact pressure points you're supposed to be targeting. It will take a little more precision when you attempt to hit the exact pressure points.

The hands' wrists are another targets. The wrists and the palm's back actually have a number of pressure points you can press, hit or hold.

At this point, you need to concentrate on attacking your wrists of your arms. A great illustration of a typical situation can be when somebody grabs you with the your collar or perhaps the moment they grasp your arms or grab your sleeves.

The hand, wrist and forearm ripe to the picking. Focus on that wrist area, particularly, where the joint of your thumb joins the wrist joint. It is possible to cut it by using the palm's edge or even the edge of your wrist.

If you strike it with enough force, it may cause the other person to let go. Also, it can cause an numbing sensation throughout his forearm. You can try the effect on your own wrist, if you wish but be careful not to pound it too in the middle.

The palm's back is home to a number of tiny bones that are quite painful when you strike them. Actually the fist of your opponent is itself a sweet place to hit. Within the art of martial of Kali the Kali have an element or a philosophy of their system of fighting called defusing the snake.

It means you take away your opponent's weapon by stopping him from engaging you during a street fight which generally involves hands, regardless of regardless of whether they're holding an weapon or not.

Find out what the typical target is - the wrists as well as the fist. The aim is to strike the wrist or hand in order to cause your opponent to release his weapon or even destroy the hand to ensure that he could not grab and use the weapon at all.

How do you go about it?

Here's a brief demonstration:

The the defensive position, with your hands in the air (like the boxer who puts his hands in a way to protect their face). Be aware that this posture is only meant to be used for training for purposes. In real-life fighting, you may not have the time needed to stand up (aka to get in the ready position) in the event of an attack. It's clear that the fist is going and it's heading right towards your face.

The opponent will make a direct left directed towards your face.

The typical reaction is to turn your back and cover yourself with your arms. This is understandable, but since you're looking to know how to defend yourself, you have to know how to defeat this reflex action.

Replace the move with a different one raise your elbow to the point that your forearm is facing over your face, and covering it to protect yourself (i.e. your forearm is parallel to your floor).

Then, point your elbow towards the fist of your opponent and then move forward after impact.

What is the result when his elbow and fist come into contact? This could cause more discomfort on his part than discomfort you feel right moment. This could lead to broken bones in the hand. It is then possible to follow up with a counter-attack or leave him in his suffering.

The Body

The torso or body contains a number of places that can be hit, and has many vital pressure points that you can hit to stop your opponent from moving. Certain areas of the torso, like the ribs , for instance are not protected at all.

Do not worry about hitting the guy in the stomach - he could have a six-pack in his abdomen, protecting the abdomen as well as other internal organs. Hit the ribs with a hammer - punch it a few times and then kick or punch it hard and with a purpose.

Another area of the body that could be your opponent. One of the areas you must aim for is your groin. You've experienced what being hit in the groin area will be like, don't you? There's no need for to see a video for it I'm sure of it. A few people are hit in the balls to the point that they vomit in pain.

Because what we're really looking for are pressure points in the body, I'd like to present to you the solar plexus. It's that section of our torso that is right here:

It's that area right above the six-pack and the point where the ribs join the abdomen. It's also known as the celiac-plexus. It does not matter what you give it, as long as you strike it with all of your strength when the opportunity arises.

You could deliver punches, strike the part you want to hit with the stick or, if your opponent is leaning backwards then you can apply an elbow on it. What is after that?

From personal experience, being hit directly in the solar plexus can cause you to stop breathing. Do you know what's under that particular patch of skin? There is no muscle or flesh layer is protecting this part.

That's your diaphragm. If you punch it, it can cause you to contract. It will cause you to stop breathing. You'll try to breathe as fast as you can, but you won't breathe until that muscle below (your diaphragm) is relaxed. If you happen to strike your trainer really intensely on that region immediately, be prepared to dial 911 and get ready to perform some artificial resuscitation . or she may need it.

Make sure to be cautious as you practice trying to hit the area.

NOTE: We've mentioned a few real pressure points in this article that could be employed in actual combat. But, what we've accomplished so far is to provide you with a list of most important targets you can use in the event you have protect yourself.

There are also other areas like the shin (give the shin a kick especially when you're wearing boots) and the knees and many more. At this point, we're going to get to the pressure points that you must apply.

Remember these areas. Hit them repeatedly with a partner in training. You can play the role of defensive player and observe how you can change angles as you attempt to hit the various targets.

In the next section, we will examine the most effective pressure points in the body to target. We will also cover the types of applications they can be utilized to help.

Chapter 9: Self Defence Scenarios And Dynamic Components Of Violence

Rear Strangle

One of the most important things to do during the midst of an assault is ensure that the attacker doesn't move behind you. If they do make an attempt to take you by the neck and you are unable to resist, then initially calm yourself and relax. The attacker may turn out to be slightly shocked by the ease of your neck. Take a step forward and grab one of his fingers, then turn it backwards in order to let the grip loosen.

Keep turning his finger as far as is possible, if he refuses to let go , and then push your elbow into the stomach as far as possible. You could even push your toes hard against his shin or foot or even poke him in the shin if you wear stilettos.

Dynamic Factors that can be found in the course of

Anger is increasing and everything in the world today can be seen as a powerful element in fighting. Sometimes, a fight occurs even though there is no reason to have one. If you are a bit smarter and applying your common sense, you will stay clear of danger and trouble for yourself.

Avoid the gangs of drunks or rowdy as much as you can. They're typically anger or jealous type who are typically discontent and are looking to get into fights. Additionally, a group of drunks has the benefit of a combined force.

Returning home in the evening is among the most problematic things, and is often the reason for can lead to fighting. Be conscious of your surroundings constantly. If someone is watching you, make sure to keep them out of sight and move to the right. Also, attempt to walk into an area that is crowded so that the attacker won't make any moves there.

The prevention of the front headlock from happening.

If an attacker attempts to strike you with the front headlock, try to first hit your arm directly into his groin. If this fails try lifting your knee to the groin. Try to release the grip of the attacker by pushing your head back and draw back your body weight.

After the front choke is put in place

Bending your elbow, and then pushing upwards is among the most effective methods to break free from the grip of your wrist. Another option to get free is to swing your arm over the attacker's body to break his grip on you, and then utilize your free hand to take on the person who is attacking you. Your movements should be effortless and your reflexes should be quick to break free from the front choke.

Escape from a headlock on the side

If the person who is attacking you with a headlock on the side from the left, grab your left hand, and then wrap it around the back of your attacker. This stops the attacker's hand from pulling down on you. Then, grab his right wrist using your right hand. Stand straight then pull the attacker's arms away.

You could even get out of from a side lock by anchoring your attacker's ankle from the back. You can also bring your attacker to the rear and then punch his head down from the front.

Another option is to grab the collar of your attacker by piercing your fingers into the throat of your attacker. You can bend a bit and then place your attacker's right leg in a cup using your right hand. Then raise his body off of the floor. Then then throw him back with great force.

Threats from a knife

If you have the option of fleeing the situation, that should be taken into consideration first. If someone comes at you with knives, it typically is a violent attack. In this instance, move toward the outside and apply both your arms , and then grab the forearm in order to lower his knife-wielding arm. Bend while doing so as you're gripping the arm that holds the knife, and it is moving toward you. After you've done this, pull the attacker's arms down by force and speed to the ground, causing him to lose balance. When you lower him you can push your left arm to his face by extending it to the side, causing injury to him.

If your attacker attempts to strike you from the bottom in a low-range attack take your hands crosswise at your wrists, then bend forward, while taking your stomach into and then strike the attacker's wrist, making it a great blocking technique.

What should you do when confronted by multiple rivals in street combat

Let's look at a frightful scenario that you've just witnessed an unimaginably entertaining college celebration. The murderer and his friends are looking around to determine whether there are witnesses to this crime And you're at the scene. What do you think you should do? Being a witness of an incident such as this puts the perpetrator in a very vulnerable position and he is attempting to turn you into the next victim. As you sit at the bar your attacker is rushing towards you in a fit of rage and is about to attack you. It is imperative to react quickly since your life is in danger! The situation doesn't seem like it's the right opportunity to talk or calm the person down, so you'll need to get down to work. Consider what's around you and the items you can use to use as weapons. You can smash him with anything like a bottle, glass or even an ash tray.

When you've found the principal person and you've already damaged the group by dealing them a huge blow. Now imagine that two buddies are still around and it's likely that they will attack you. You can see who darts at you first. Then, you can give him with a punch that knocks him out of his mind for a minimum of a couple of minutes. Utilize the ducking movement when a third party is at you. Then, look at the exit points, and then make your escape prior to any members of the group show on you!

If this scenario could happen in reality you must prepare a game plan for your actions. Your body posture is the most crucial aspect. Do not turn your back towards your opponent. Be conscious of you surroundings. make sure to practice these strategies every single day. It's not about being fearful but simply being aware to ensure that, when the time comes, you'll be prepared, just because you've prepared beforehand.

Things to keep in mind when facing numerous attackers:

Your mental battle is just equally important as your physical battle, in fact, it's even more crucial! A positive and calm attitude affects the physical fight to the max.

Determine the leader of the group and then bring him first, so as to dissuade other members of the group

Make a mental game with your adversaries by breaking the strong connection in the group, which could be a different person from the leader.

One serious and obvious harm to any member of the group may deter the confidence of the entire group together.

The goal is to weaken the group in every way whether by attacking a primary member, or by having a one or more side kicks or to that break up the group.

Do not use boring and predictable techniques. Find new ways to perform to be able to be awed by the attacker and his entire team.

Chapter 10: Learn to Maintain Control Over Your Energy Levels

Synopsis

In the realm of self-defense strategies for psychics You will be able to see that there are specific methods to manage the intensity of your energy in complete control. To achieve this you need to follow these things:

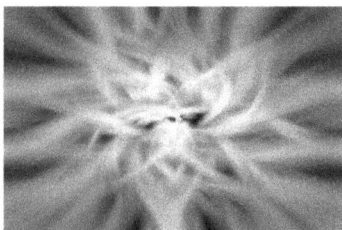

Check It Out Carefully

Mundane - You have to help the person get from a habitual mindset and to a common and everyday perspective. It is important to ask the individual what he or she was doing the previous day. It is also possible to ask questions , such as if they're happy with their boss, or what colors they like best.

* Shielding - Create energy shields around a person to stop energy flow, which can create issues. If someone is incapable of creating their individual shield, they may create it for them temporarily.

* Blocking is similar to shielding but it focuses more in the physical sense. You must place yourself in a physical space between your self and the thing that your the source of your distress is. Blocking has the benefit by shielding yourself from the physical obstacles caused by the blocking power that supports you.

* Charging can boost the energy levels of an individual by putting energy into their body.

* Re-turning, it's when you return the energy of a person to a higher vibrational level to handle the greater energy level, without causing harm.

* Energy-shifting is exactly the same as returning, but at a momentary and smaller scale. It can alter the frequency of vibration of a person , temporarily greater or lesser for a specified time just.

Find the Equilibrium Your energy will search for and find its equilibrium on its own. This is called equilibrium. It is all about letting your body relax in order to let more energy flow into and out of your body without having to exert it. This method is also beneficial for those looking to find harmony with the surrounding.

Breaking connections the energy threads may be created during your work routine or by magic. This usually happens when you're not aware. If you cut off this connection physically or emotionally and you are unable to find the cause of your issue is a lot easier to achieve.

* Regaining focus - reminding you to pay attention to something that demands you to return to the place you are.

* Stilling is the method of moving your body into a calm stable, calm, and peaceful state. It is the physical sequence of balancing, tuning and finding your center.

* Centering - This approach can be useful in situations where you lack the focus on something. This is the psyche-based method of balancing, stilling and tuning.

The Balancing can help you make your energy levels balance. It's similar to equilibrium, but you are able to utilize it when you can't relax enough to achieve equilibrium. The equilibrium can be found and allow your energy to flow freely.

* Attuning - connect with your soul's core. This is the spiritual aspect of the process of balancing, stilling, and re-centering.

Closing - in order to manage your energy level it is recommended to shut down the chakras of the person for a short period of time. You can do this in part or completely. This method will assist you to stop the flow of energy into and out of that individual.

* Cocooning - creating a bubble or shield of energy around someone. This can be used to remove individuals from your energy circle but without realizing of what you've done.

* Relaxing - there are instances that people require breaks. This can allow you

to boost the current amount of energy. A brief nap and enough rest will allow your body and help you to gain more energy.

* Remaining present is the list of skills that can be used to identify the sensation that you've lost control of your body by channeling or possession. Learn to be aware of the warning signs such as trace states, body movements that are impulsive and the ability to sense thoughts, feelings and voices that are not really from you.

* Shock - A surprising feeling or sound could break an individual from the place where the attention of the person is not present. A loud noise close to you, like a snarling hand clap will generally bring someone back from an altered situation. At some point in the event that the situation is very serious, physical actions like slapping the face an attack on the shin

could return a person right and without any long-term or permanent adverse consequences. These should be utilized only as a last resort, and it is recommended to apply this technique under certain circumstances only.

* Radial grounding - these are the strategies can be used to get rid of all the energy within a person. They include physical and even more than the energetic movements. A good example is an heel drop. The person should jump, before he/she reaches the ground, request for him/her to lock their knees and then to landing hard with both the heels. The body will jar when you land, since the energy will be pushed into the ground and away.

* Grounding is the final method can be used to increase your energy level, but it is also regarded as the most commonly used method. It's suggested to be utilized in all

situations, but this is usually not the right method to use. If you are suffering from low energy levels, this method may not be the most effective option for your particular situation. If you're suffering from energy imbalance or blockage the technique won't be beneficial for you. If you are trying to increase your energy levels, this method is likely to draw the energy from your body. In order to make yourself "mobile" as well as "fluid" grounded, it can affect the process and will ensure that you remain rooted. It's only beneficial in the event that you are able to resist some thing. In most cases, you can do some magic and then reflect that energy without intention behind it. This way, you'll gain the benefit of not having to deal with the energy, however it is crucial to keep this in mind as a goal.

As you will observe, there are many strategies you can employ to manage your energy level. These techniques will enable you to improve your ability to control your inner part to help you focus better on the outside. Being in control of your energy is part of your psyche's defense strategy.

Chapter 11: The Spaces That Are Open Spaces Or Transitional Spaces

"Open Spaces" or transitional spaces are spaces which allow an ambushable or escape for attackers[5[5]. These spaces are open and easily accessible/transitional with open doors at all times including, but not limited to, moments like walking down the street, waiting for bus or elevator, at a gas station, shopping, withdrawing money from an ATM, walking on the pavement. In the sense that these are public and social spaces.

If you find yourself in these areas, be cautious. Keep your purse closed or count your cash etc. Pay attention to more. Always be aware of what's happening before and surrounding you. It is possible to use windows in the building or mirrors, in the event that they exist or shiny surfaces to observe what's in front of you. Don't be distracted by your phone, but remain aware of your surroundings. Make sure you don't block your ears, a crucial sense organ when you listen to music through headphones. Make sure you can see ahead when you close your eyes, which are the most vital sense organ on a cellphone.

It can also be improved awareness by not being in solitude and being when you are in an open space. Awareness is essential when you're in an open area! You can be sure that none of those people that walked through the normal places of the course of a normal day, and then were attacked, thought it was the end of the morning of their lives. they awoke in early morning.

Be aware of the surroundings when you enter your car . Lock the doors when you are inside. Keep the doors of your car secured at all times. Secure the doors even when you need to conduct an unimportant errand. For instance, if you leave your car at a petrol station, or buy something at the market or from a hawker ensure that you close the doors. This safeguards you from assaults but also stops carjacking and theft.

We've now covered the abundance of spaces as well as the importance of being aware, it's crucial to distinguish between paranoia and awareness. A habit of being aware can help you to spend your time more effectively efficient, productively and maybe pleasant. The brain is trained to be aware, and awareness can save lives.

Situational Awareness

The goal for now is to establish "Situational awareness" in transitional zones. Situational Awareness allows us to see with a keen eye on what's going on around us, and to be more mindful of people and objects. It also allows us to assess the situation and identify potential threats. This includes using our senses and instincts.

For example, if we see someone in an icy helmet or a snow-mask during a hot day it will occur to us that something's not quite right. When we hear in the opposite direction of us when walking on the streets and become more alert, we should be aware. If someone's coming directly towards us, and there are strangers around us or staring at us watching us, and, most important of all when they're holding knives, choppers or screwdriver, you should be aware of sharp objects , etc. ....For this it is important to develop the habit of watching (even even if it's you are not asking) anyone who is who is approaching you. Be aware of all.

Indeed, one of the most crucial skills to develop in your life is knowing who and what is risky for us and also to discern between good and evil. Awareness buys you time until a threat-danger-attacker reaches your intimate zone in case of a possible attack, and time in turn allows you to make plans on how to evade a threat[6].

Farnum's Law: Rules of Stupid

Rules of stupid will remind you of the lessons from your childhood, such as be a decent person, not going to wrong places, and not to make bad friends, etc. Below, we will look at the rules of stupid set out by Farnum[77

1.Don't visit dangerous locations, (don't go to unnecessary dangerous locations)

2.Don't spend time with naive people (don't be with bad people or avoid going out with strangers or people who aren't trustworthy)

3.Don't leave at unsuitable times (i.e. don't go out after midnight unless you have to)

4.Don't make a mess of things (stay away from harmful dangerous, harmful or unnecessary things)

If you violate one of the four (four) rules listed above, even if everything is well in the event of an unlikely situation when you break at least two rules it means you're in danger!

Ambush and Alert

If you have your honor, property, or your property are the target of a criminal is likely to be targeted and savagely attacked. Ambush can occur in different ways.

In one kind attack, the attacker(s) locate a suitable position and remain in open spaces of transitional space. This is referred to as "Positional ambush". In this instance it is carried out immediately and without prior preparation by the attacker. The attacker pounces on you directly and then commits an armed robbery or an attack of some kind. Be aware in these instances because there is only a brief period between the moment of intention as well as the moment of actual assault.

Another kind of ambush is "Normalcy Ambush" which is described in the subject "Underestimation". Someone who is not familiar with you may walk up to you and pretend to be talking on the phone . Or the attacker may approach like he's going to ask a question. They may also smile. You wouldn't be in a position to keep your eyes on him. Everything looks quite normal. He then shows you his knife, gun or a similar tool of intimidation/threat[8] and demands your money or property. The threat could be to force you to another location with malicious intent. In this scenario it is important to ensure your privacy. You may see the attack coming based on the attitudes of an attacker and with the help of the cues explained in "Pre-Attack Indicators/Pre-Attack Cues" and consequently prevent any such attack, make a counter attack or best of all, you may give a slip and escape.

Random and unpredictable attacks

It is important to note that certain types of attacks are inevitably attacks, regardless of the level of your awareness. In some instances, you could be attacked at the most inconvenient time or in the most inconvenient area, or in an surprising way. For instance, a piece of equipment falling from a height when you're walking on the sidewalk or a vehicle moving towards you when you're walking across the street. It can be difficult to maintain concentration in large crowds. In these situations prepare yourself to handle what happens after an attack i.e. remain calm, avoid fainting or freezing, display resistance and plan your escape and learn basic first-aid techniques for your loved ones and yourself.

Random attacks are committed by morbid, demon-possessed people without any sign of attack, nor verbal assaults that are completely normal. The attacker arrives and attacks at random. There are few indicators prior to attack and zero in such attacks. Sometimes, the attacker will pose a question that isn't quite right to get close, only to reverse and attack. This is known as"the creep alarm..

Being aware of the possibility of falling victimization is essential for attacks. We must avoid shutting our eyes with mobile phones and other similar devices. Particularly, it is possible to escape or avoid due to our enhanced physical abilities. It's difficult to defend ourselves from these evil individuals[9 or their attacks. It is imperative to pray that Allah [10to protect us from these types of people.

Vulnerable Population

Life isn't stable, and it changes constantly. Every living thing enters the life, becomes disabled or sick, and then becomes old. Then each living thing dies at some point. We might not always be strong and healthy all the time. The elderly and children, as well as the mentally and physically disabled women and men are considered to be vulnerable populations that are more likely to be targeted as they are weak, defenseless and vulnerable, and have less capacity to defend themselves[11].

In light of the negative impact of moral depravity and moral corruption on our society, we need to be extra vigilant to not fall victim. We see in the media and on television the plight of depraved people and that's just the top of the ocean.

The requirement for self-defense techniques is especially important for those in need and their dependent relatives. As one ages or is diagnosed with illness, mental and physical abilities diminish and, consequently, more focus should be paid to certain abilities, especially those that deal with awareness of distance, margin and awareness. People should be vigilant about their own space and distances. If they can they should carry tear gas or firearms (however gun ownership is not a good idea in the US). They should also think about the use and use of the tools described by "Force Multipliers". Children must always be taught to maintain an appropriate distance from strangers. The need for supervision and limits is imperative throughout the places where they are permitted to travel on their own.

The most vulnerable group especially children considers adults to be incredibly strong and invincible. But, it might be possible to quickly break away from the grasp of an adversary by a sudden, painful pain. escape techniques, or even cause alarm by shouting and fleeing from the scene.

In the event incident of an assault, in the event that an innocent bystander, accompanied by someone from a vulnerable population (senior relative, children, etc.) (for instance, if you're at the site of a robbery, or a street fight when you are shopping in the market) Don't be a spectator and just be a spectator. You and your spouse should take your child and quickly leave the incident. If you're unable to do that, then go to a safe place. Make sure to contact the police!

Chapter 12: What If I Fail?

Life is full of ups and downs, however we need to learn to not take them in our own mind. Whatever amount of you think about it, we cannot guarantee physical victory, but we can guarantee that we will win in our minds! In all the years I instructing self-defense classes for women, this is a subject we have to be aware of.

How will I cope if do lose?

It is the first thing to do not to internalize the experience. I have a beloved friend who I had to go up through ranks during my early years who stated that he was the best person to lose an opponent that he ought to have defeated. "I might lose but he didn't defeat me." This should be the mindset we adopt throughout our lives for everything! When you train your mind in the right way and devote time to your self image, losing becomes much easier to handle! Even when serious injuries are in the mix. Always remember that there's no shame in seeking help!

You will only lose if the idea of losing be an integral part of your life!

The society of today

If you consider the state of society today and consider the information you just read you'll begin to understand the reasons. The reason why people do not take action is simple. They don't realize that they are suffering. When you consider the current victim-strike mentality and the level of depression people are suffering from. It is easy to identify the root cause behind the problems. There's always a root reason! Particularly when the numbers are this high! However, the reason why people aren't able to examine this is that it places the burden of responsibility on your on your shoulders. Nobody can be a as a victim when this happens.

It is likely to be evident in your life what your most prevalent thoughts are even if you do not remember them. Let's take a look at an example from our lives. There are eight people at an unlit street corner eager to get across. There are two people at each corner. A car crash occurs at the intersection of the roads. Police are called. Every person who witnessed the incident, if asked independently, will give an entirely different story of the incidents. Whyis that? Because they'll think of the incident as something that their subconscious mind associates with. If they were involved in a car accident , their perception will be affected because of that accident. They're not lying, it's the way we operate.

As an additional illustration

* If you feel you are being targeted due to race, you'll encounter more resentment.

* If you're scared of spiders, then you'll encounter more spiders

* If you're concerned about a new bad relationship and you end up in a negative relationship.

If you believe you're a skilled martial artist, you'll discover other martial artists to study from.

* If you think that money is simple to earn You will make plenty of it.

If you think that it is difficult to earn money then you are probably poor.

It is applicable to all aspects of life, regardless of whether you want it or you don't. The process of fixing this can be a long process and that's not a negative thing! It's just something that we must be able to conquer. To conquer ourselves is the most crucial!

The best athletes do this even though they don't even realize that they do it! It's all you have to do is watch them speak to get the idea.

This is the research of self-improvement. It's so simple and is simple even if you think so! However, you have to be alert and be diligent!

You can be successful too!

Making the Self-Image

Making a positive self image isn't difficult or easy. It is dependent on the individual and their motivation to make positive changes. There are examples every day of "poor" self-images everywhere you look. People fight over things that aren't important. People getting "offended" simply by words! In reality, they are seeking reasons to be offended since they are what they think of themselves as! "I am victimized by "this" "that" as well as"the "other things." What's required is a deep look within to find out the beliefs that are forming them and then begin to alter them.

The thing that is truly sad is that our business that is the martial arts field is one of the most infamous cases of poor self-image and yet we are expected to build "self self-esteem." It's an incredible failure from our side!

How many times have you attended events that an "master" is trying to place himself or herself over the other participants? You may have read about "watch dogs" groups that discuss the person who is a fraud or this person who is running an McDojo. This is kind of absurd, isn't? Recently I encountered a problem that involved a well-known and respected master who was trying to continually show how important he is instead of just taking in the moment.

What others think about you is not your concern! This is among the most difficult things for people to comprehend. Your opinion of me or my work, is yours! Yes, I'm trying to get you purchase my books and follow my instructions however if you choose not do so, it's on you, not me! A lot of people will be able to reject the message rather than take it on board! If enough people reject it, I should review the content and possibly bring it back! Do not feel guilty about myself and quit!

Everyone has their own unique self-image, and we all have to improve their self-image every day! Everyone needs to speak to ourselves more positively and take care of ourselves better, and take care of ourselves. If we can do this, we'll see a dramatic transformation in the world that surrounds us!

Chapter 13: Tools at Your Disposition

Bystander Intervention

Abel Christianson heard the cry for help in the distance as he was returning back home from a party at the college on a cool Wisconsin night. He quickly stepped forward to meet the co-ed student as well as unidentified male. She was begged to return back to her family. In spite of all the efforts made by her father who tried to convince Abel that everything is fine but he was aware of the dangers. Abel who was an athlete was not letting up and was not walking away. He rushed to help her up and took back to her bedroom until she was secure with her family.

Abel has never seen this woman before however, he didn't need to get to know her. He was already aware of right from wrong. This is the foundation of Bystander Intervention and men who take their responsibility. The responsibility is for themselves, others, and for the safety of the community.

In recent times, there has been a desire to involve people to prevent sexual assaults. This year's Campus Sexual Violence Elimination Act was an important factor in this, since it required that universities educate students on how to prevent sexual assault.

The purpose of any intervention is to engage the most allies you can to prevent sexual assaults. It's all about the character of your student community and every individual who has been a victim. When students realize that they are the kind of person who can intervene in a fight that causes a dramatic shift. They recognize that it's no longer acceptable to remain at the sidelines. It's not a reality show.

The programs have proven that they are extremely effective in reducing the number of assaults. It is difficult to find concrete numbers get, however due to the fact that it can be difficult to quantify an assault that never occurred.

Schools are able to offer these courses on the internet and in person. There are benefits to both alternative.

Online training permits a wider spread over a realistic timeframe. The research conducted by the National Center for Biotechnology Information shows that this method can maintain its effectiveness for a year.

In-person training is believed to be more effective in reaching out to the public since many students are used to learning in person.

Intervention training is crucial and require your help. However, there's an issue. We have no control over others and their reactions or react to an event. The rest of the chapter is focused on the tools within our control. Make sure you check out the resource page for an amazing group of people working using interventions.

Situational Awareness

It is believed that 80percent of plane crashes were the result of human mistakes[8[8]. In reports of aviation accidents post-accident you'll see phrases like lack of awareness frequently. The same awareness of the situation that requires to keep an aircraft in the air is the same level of awareness we employ to stay out of dangers in situations. The concept of situational awareness is divided into three distinct parts.

The components are perception, comprehension , and visual. Let's look at an example. If you are walking along the road in the summer heat and you see that there's a man standing in front of you with a long trench coat and his face covered with an athletic cap. He's getting ready go into the same building that you are in.

Perception lets you see your surroundings and assess the various components and the overall impact of the surroundings. We know that the man does not fit into the environment. Comprehensiveness allows us to put the latest information with our previous experiences and reach the conclusion that he's likely hiding something, perhaps a weapon. Visualization, also known as projection, helps us see the various possibilities for how the situation might unfold.

In this moment, we must decide and take action. What do you think?

Cooper's Color Codes is a commonly employed tool for indicating different levels of awareness in law enforcement agencies and military.

*White indicates a normal baseline. When you're at back at home with your family your guard is off and you're at peace.

The color yellow is generally thought to refer to the level you are at when in public area. You are aware of people and to the surrounding.

*Orange means that you've identified a potential threat, and you're contemplating ways to get back to yellow. This could mean that you're leaving the area, or they are.

*Red means go. There is a threat, and you fight or flee response will kick in. Take action now!

Keep in mind that the aim isn't a perpetual condition of fear. You'll be exhausted and feel awkward in social situations. Also, it's not logical, but you're less likely to be calm and recognize dangers when you're hyped up out in public. The most important thing to remember is to pay attention to certain things or people who make you uncomfortable.

Action Steps

1.When you're walking around or in a space take note of the objects around you that could serve as weapons to defend yourself.

2.Practice detailing your environment. How many people are there in the room? What colour shirt are they wearing? What number of hats are there present in the room? It might seem unnecessary to be aware of such details however, it's all about routine. You're probably not aware of the number of hats on the table, will not make a difference to your life. But taking the time focus on the small details could save your life.

Fear and Adrenaline

Uncertainty and fear are common in times of conflict. If there is fear, there is adrenaline. The majority of athletes are used to small doses of adrenaline that help fight the pain, speed up their runs or leap higher during the final seconds in the final seconds. The adrenaline rush is different. It is a rush of adrenaline that can be felt instantly and is a result of fear but it's for our advantage.

My closest friends are aware that I'm an nerd, and also a huge Dr. Who fan. There's a moment during the show, Listen of Dr. Who that resonates with me because of its totally precise description of the fear. It is in the scene that the main Dr. Who, The Doctor, is going on a new adventure. He meets the young boy who is scared of the things that lie beneath his mattress.

Dr. Who, after gaining many insights from his journeys, takes the boy from the side and informs him that fear can be a good thing. Incredulous, the boy turns at the screen and is attentive.

Dr.Who: "Want to know the reason why this is good? I'll tell you how the fear in your eyes. Your heart is beating fast, I feel it through your fingers. A lot of blood and oxygen moving through your brain. It's like rocket fuel. Now, you're able to accelerate faster, you'll be able to push more vigorously, and you can leap higher than you have ever before you've ever done. And because you're so alert it's as if you reduce the speed of your life. What's wrong with being afraid? The ability to be scared is a superpower. This is your power. There's a danger in this space And do you know who it is? You are the one who is at risk!"

The rush of adrenaline you feel from fear will increase your gross motor abilities. In this sense, these are activities such as swinging, running, and more. They do not require coordination with smaller muscles. In general it's very good. These are the factors which significantly increase your capability to live by making us resilient as nails.

But, our motor skills suffer. One of the most popular known motifs from Hollywood might be the fright scene in which the bad guy is chased by his victims through the (insert random setting) and they finally reach their front door. They open the door, and keys are moving in their hands Then boom. They throw away the keys. The sprint through the doors was pure adrenaline-fuelled gross muscle with large muscles. The coordination required to open the door by inserting the key that's about 8.8 millimeters high into the keyhole that's barely taller, it's fine motor.

Action Steps

Experience is the most important factor in making your adrenaline work for you. It's possible to have the experience but if you're not taking the steps to put that knowledge into practice by taking action, what's the purpose? To get your adrenaline flowing and increase your energy levels, you must practice an authentic self-defense system like Krav Maga. There are a variety of options however Krav Maga focuses on training that challenges you physically by focusing on gross motor actions, and won't take an entire decade to learn.

How can training help you become acclimated to the adrenaline rush? Consider it as if you were driving an automobile. When you first drove in a car, you felt that the controls seemed foreign and unwieldy, the car moved more quickly than you thought. It's likely that your parents and you were anxious. You might have thought that you'd never get grasp of this.

With repetition, consistency and perseverance, we are able to control our speed and potential of the car. The driving on the highway, which was previously an intense, exhausting and stressful experience, is now a routine task. Both the car and the road will changes. Our perceptions and abilities to deal with it, alter. Understanding the fundamentals of self-defense at a reputable center is similar. With training, you learn to manage your body's response to adrenaline. You're no longer an uninvolved participant in the ride. You have an input into the direction you travel.

A companion video is available that is included in the book. It's not as if it is a replacement for the actual thing, but rather as an excellent starting point. The information and training that is provided in this book are a panacea. There is nothing better than finding a place to learn and get your hands sweaty. If you venture out in the world to discover a place where you can learn self-defense, these are some of the qualities you must look for in the training facility:

*The methods must be simple enough to be effective even when you're scared with a heart rate of near 200 beats per minute. This means that they must include movements that are gross in nature.

It can make you feel uncomfortable. Training should push you out of your comfort zone to the point that you feel challenged but not to the point that you are overwhelmed.

*Safety is always a factor. If safety concerns appear to be taking a back seat to the activity, get go away immediately.

The devil is in the particulars. It is essential that they spend the time to explain what they are doing when they are demonstrating something to you. What is the reason they perform the actions they do? It's important.

A good self-defense course covers more than just how to punch and kick. It will teach you the fundamentals like self-defense laws and situational awareness. You will also learn the right time to leave.

Finding out what type of style is the best self-defense. one that is an unintentional path to take and is can be counterproductive. It's usually down to the person. If you have specific questions on finding a training location, you can email me at Andre.jherbert@gmail.com.

Fight, Fight or Freeze

The two most well-known reactions to an adrenaline-inducing situation are flight or fight. Fighting is fairly straightforward. You recognize the dangerand take the threat head-on using any weapon you're equipped with. There is always an improvised weapon in the vicinity. Keep in mind that our sole goal is to fight for long enough to be able to escape and not be the champion.

A flight response is usually the most effective option. It's not an issue in the event that you are able to get out safely. It's that the only thing that counts. Our eyes are located in the in front of us and not on the sides like predators, but keep in mind that we can be prey by choice. Even big cats suffer from an failure rate of between 90% and 95 percent in the wilderness, when hunting an animal on their own. Flight response is a good thing.

The freeze response is the most hazardous choice of all three. The freeze reaction is the one you do not wish to trigger. We are wired to either fight or flee to escape; these are the options which will bring us safely home. We can either fight to the point that the predator realizes that we're not the victim, and we escape. We also run away from the danger before it has the chance to be overwhelming us. The freeze response makes us like a deer caught in the headlights.

If we are faced with the necessity to make a choice the most dangerous option is to not make a decision. There are many instances of instances where this principle is being played out. What happens if you do not respond to your professor's requests for a conference? What happens if you freeze and do not notice that mole on your arm instead of visiting the doctor?

Teddy Roosevelt said it best with this quote from his mic drop:

"In every moment, you have to make a decision. The most effective option is to do the right thingto do, the next best thing to do is the wrong option and the worst option is to do nothing."

Truth is I am unable to give you, in any circumstance, the best solution for you at this moment. It is you who are the sole person on earth who has to make that decision in the face of an attack. If you decide to fight, do it with a vengeance. If you choose flight, don't look back.

The option of freezing is one, but not one we would like to choose. A good mental model will be crucial to avoid the possibility of a freeze reaction.

Mental modeling

Our brain is a powerful computer that is capable of complex calculations. We often don't realize how many calculations and recalculations we are required to perform each minute of every day. The most remarkable abilities of the human mind is the ability to imagine things that aren't real.

The process of mental modeling can be a technique employed by athletes, CEOs and special operations teams to assist them in creating an outline of the possibilities.

The CEO could imagine how changes to policies will positively or negatively impact the business in the coming six, 12, and 24 months.

Before a big game the basketball player might imagine how they will begin the game. From the first moments of the ball all the way through the fourth quarter, when they are at the free-throw line to hit the winning basket of the game.

As a security guard You should think about what would happen in the event that you go on the run and a danger approaches you. What are your options? What are you going to say? Are they threatening or simply a person seeking directions? This is the reason mental modeling is essential in preventing freezing in times of danger.

If you've never thought about being attacked and how to react, your reaction are likely to be slow, similar to computers processing too much information. It will take longer reacting than executing because your brain isn't used to this kind of scenario.

Our brains have a hard discernment between the real and the imagined, and that is exactly why top performers make use of it. They've seen the path toward success inside their heads and they've planned for it. The reality they see is similar to the reality they've seen before.

It does not have to be a sad issue where the majority of our time is spent imagining someone attacking us. We are aware of what can happen when you drop your phones, therefore we purchase an iPhone case without even a second thought. It's more valuable than your phone.

Action Steps

Every day, when you're out in public, perform an exercise in thought. You can ask yourself a few what-if questions.

Would you act What would you do if:

*You're enjoying your night out and someone walks in and is threatening one of your friends.

You heard gunshots coming from the hall, which direction would you flee to?

There was a fire that was extinguished by the primary exit.

*You enter the Uber taxi, but the driver immediately switches off the phone and GPS, and then drives off the track.

The body is not able to move where the mind has never been. Craft your action plan for several scenarios unique to your life. Your plan will put you in the best possible position to survive.

Chapter 14: Understanding Strength Training

If you are a possible grappler is required to build your power. You should be able to take on your adversaries, remain well-balanced, and to withstand any force or force acting on your. Strength, aside from endurance is the most crucial ability to possess which will become the sole one covered in this book.

There are numerous misconceptions regarding strength training. One of them is that it is only performed by those who wish to build muscle. It's not the complete picture. Lifting weights is a simple way to build strength this is the reason it's called strength training. It allows you to get more prepared to handle the weight of heavy objects and resist heavier forces.

Before we begin in this chapter, it is crucial to be aware that exercise can reduce calories, and therefore is difficult if you aren't in good condition. Don't be compelled to perform every single thing in this chapter in a hurry. We have discussed in the chapter, each person has a unique percentage of muscle fibers. If you're not able to maintain the pace of the exercises included in this section, you are welcome to lower the intensity, and then gradually increase the intensity until you are able to keep up.

Strength and cardio

Cardio, which is short for cardiovascular exercise, refers to any kind of exercise that your heart rate increases for a set amount of time. Examples include cycling or running.

Many people train for their cardio due to the belief that it will help people lose weight. Although this is true, it's an oversimplified. It is possible to skip all cardio and still lose weight, provided that you eat a healthy diet and are exercising regularly. In addition, contrary to what is commonly believed, aerobic exercise won't diminish the strength gains of your muscles.

The main reason to exercise is to improve fitness levels for your cardio. It lets you stay longer in your exercise which is an excellent indicator of endurance. This is due to the fact that you are working to produce greater levels of energy for an extended period of time.

There aren't any negative consequences when you combine cardio with strengthening exercises. While you are able to build for strength on your own without having to exercise I suggest you split your time between doing a particular program. You should only do cardio every once in a while. This will make you stay longer and be more effective at grappling.

It doesn't matter which kind of cardio you wish to engage in. All you need to do is to keep increasing intensities of the workout in order to achieve outcomes. Every session, begin with a warm-up with a low intensity. This allows your body to adapt to the exercise and aid in avoiding injury.

Basic terminology

When it comes to discussing the subject of strength training there are some essential terms that need to be clarified since they are used in every situation. The following terms are:

1. Intensity. This was already previously mentioned. Intensity is the energy level you're putting into.

2. Rep or repetition. A rep is the time you've completed the exercise correctly

and completely. exercise. For instance, if are able to complete three sit-ups in a row, you've completed 3 repetitions.

3. Set. A set is an assortment of repetitions. Training typically takes three sets with 8-12 reps for each set.

4. Form. Form is the term used to describe your posture or the way you execute a specific exercise. If you are not properly formed, it will result in negative results, and expose you to a greater risk of injuries.

5. Dumbbell. A dumbbell is small bar that has weights to strengthen one arm. It is not to be confused with barbells.

6. Barbell. Barbells are a bar that is long and has adjustable weights designed to strengthen both arms simultaneously.

How do you build strength?

We have now reviewed the most fundamental terms of strength training, I'll talk about how you can begin strengthening your body.

The first thing to do is perform your warm-up prior to each exercise. For this, you must do one set of the exercises you'll be performing with no weights. This will build your muscles for the exercises to follow.

The most effective type of strength-training program is one that uses compound moves. What that means is that the repetitions are used to can be used to strengthen two or more joints simultaneously. They are more beneficial for overall muscle development instead of focusing on developing muscles at specific points. Additionally, they help your workout more efficient as you work multiple muscles at each time. In addition, since isolated exercises aren't as strong as those in real life the compound movement gives you an opportunity to train more realistically and be prepared for real-life circumstances.

Another thing to figure out is that strength training demands a an enormous amount of lifting weight. It is only possible to improve your muscles if you notice that you're unable to finish 10 reps with the same weight. This means that you're really working your muscles and are getting used to lifting heavier weights.

This is a well-known beginner's program that will surely yield positive results if you follow it regularly. The program is known as "Starting Strength" You are required to complete a set of exercises every day, which is three times each week.

There are two lists of workouts that you must complete. You must complete one list first and the second one next time. Be sure to select the most intense weight. In this exercise, you should employ that same amount of weight in each set of a particular exercise. Be aware that these are exercises for compound muscles. While they focus on specific areas in your body, these exercises target your other muscles too. You'll be able to see your arms strengthen even if your next workouts are not focused on your arms.

Workout A:

3 sets x 5 reps barbell squat. The basic idea behind the barbell squat is to place the barbell with your shoulders while the knees are bent in an squat. This workout will strengthen your quadriceps or muscles that are located in side of your legs. The form is crucial in this exercise.

To perform the barbell squat, place the barbell on the rack above your chest. Then, position yourself in a way your barbell will be held by your back shoulders. Keep the bar in place. When you're ready, remove the bar from the floor and sit up straight. Then, bend your hips and your knees to the side in order to sit down. Be sure that your knees and your legs are pointed towards exactly the same direction. Make sure you do not bend your back. Continue to bend till your legs are in line with the floor. Bring your knees back and return to the original position. This is just one repetition.

To add additional information to the form, make sure to focus on the forward direction while keeping your foot straight. This will help you keep your balance and even out the barbell's weight.

3 x 5 bench press. The bench press requires you to raise the barbell while lying down, face down, on the bench. The

exercise is primarily focused on your chest or pectorals.

To perform a bench presses lay down on the bench, face-up and take the barbell off the rack while keeping your grips in a wide space from one another. Place the barbell on your chest, then lower it. Then push it back up to ensure your arms remain completely stretched out. This is a single rep.

1 x 5 deadlift. Deadlifting involves bending your knees while holding the barbell, and then stand straight. This workout strengthens your gluteus maximus, which is the muscle located at the bottom of your body.

For a deadlift, stand straight and flat on your feet. The barbell should be placed on the floor , just above your feet. Squat down and grasp the barbell with your the shoulder's length. Straighten up by extending your hips and knees. Reposition your shoulders when doing this. Restore the barbell to the floor with the squat movement.

Like the barbell squat form is crucial for deadlifts. Make sure that your hips remain low and your shoulders are elevated while your back and arms are straight. Make sure you don't shift the position of your knees or your legs. Keep the barbell in close proximity to your body and draw the weight towards you. You may find the use of gym chalk may assist in strengthening your grip.

2 dips 5-8. Dips require a specific apparatus that has bars extended. It is a simple exercise that requires you to stand up and lower yourself down and over while lifting those legs to the back. Don't swing your body upwards; it's cheating. If you discover that you're too light and you

can easily perform more than 8 reps per set, you should wear an adjustable belt that weighs so that you'll be heavier.

Workout B:

3 x 5 barbell squat. It is similar to one from Workout A.

3 5 standing press. This workout strengthens your shoulders. Standing military presses require you to raise the barbell above the top of your head and stand.

To accomplish this, put the barbell on the rack at the level of your chest. Take the barbell by hand looking forward, and a space larger that your shoulder. Knees should be bent and you can place your barbell in the middle that your neck bone. Lift the bar and hold it for a couple of minutes. Lower it down towards your neck bone. This is a single rep.

3 x 5 Pendlay rows. This workout trains the back muscles. The Pendlay Row is similar to a deadlift, with the exception the frame is bent inwards, and you're squatting. This will require your back muscles to perform.

To perform, place your feet on the floor, flat while bending your knees a bit to create an Squat. The barbell should be held at your shoulders' width, then raise the bar toward you stomach, until the shoulders of your in line with the floor. Then, return the barbell to the ground. This is one rep.

Be sure that your posture is correct by making sure that your knees, feet and hips are always aligned and your back does not bend.

2 5 chin-ups x 2. Like the dips, it requires you to push your entire body upwards to the point that your head is over the bar you're using. If you feel that you are too

heavy, try an adjustable belt that is weighted.

The following workout routine will help you get started to build your strength. Once you're at ease with a specific weight, you should always try to lift more weights. This will aid you become a master grappler, just like Milo from Croton.

Does stretching help me?

This chapter will conclude with a brief discussion about stretching. A lot of people use stretching to warm up. It is believed that it helps relax your muscles, preventing soreness following your exercise. But this isn't the situation. Stretching before exercise actually tightens muscles and increases the likelihood of injuries.

However, stretching isn't necessarily bad. You can stretch out after your exercise. It will also aid in improving posture and along with exercises for the back, is recommended for people suffering from scoliosis.

Chapter 15: Self Defense for Teenage Age Girls and Young Women If You Have to Take on a Sexually Attempted Intruder!

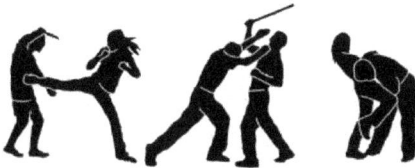

Females and females alike tune and these self-defense techniques and advice can save your life. The majority of sexual assaults or assaults are committed by girls and women aged between 16 and 26 years old. The statistics are alarming for assaults around 1 in 4 females will have been assaulted at some point in your lifetime. Of the rapes they are responsible for 77% of victims knew the perpetrator.

This means that the person who is likely to target you may be a male family member or male friend or even a sweetheart of a mother or sister or even a date attack. Don't let yourself become a victim, never. Take a look at this article, and give it to everyone you know to ensure to be able to survive and also assist someone else.

The most important thing you need to do is to be prepared. Every environment can represent a potential target so be aware. Be aware of WHO is in your vicinity. Let me retell this to you! The victim could also be male relative don't assume to be protected, despite the fact that you're isolated from the rest of the family by the father of your friend's partner that you will be protected in the event you're on the couch in your bra and underwear or you have just got into the bath at their house. The majority of sexual stalkers or attackers are opportunistic by nature. They are looking for an opportunity and jump on the opportunity, but they realize that they aren't going to be caught. Sexual predators or attackers is betting on the humiliation of you and humiliation. you'll be reluctant to talk about it. NEWS Streak! If you're brave enough and decide to speak about your ideas, it is likely that you are not going to be considered in any way! This is your oath to his. What if we suppose that you are a more mature and well-known, distinguished man, in the unlikely possibility that anyone believes that to be true and accepts that you took it and you were able to resist to sexually entice him.

Because this happened previously to me by a male family member I'm going to tell you that nobody trusted me also. Even if I don't know who you are, I believe that this has was your experience and may be the case for your friend too. Now I'll provide you with some self-defense techniques to pound your adversary on the _____!

Every minute that passes from today and continuing into the near future, I want you to be more conscious of where you areand who you are and envision a situation that any part of the tools can be used for your defense. First of all, don't give open access to the sick! Don't hide, and don't reveal everything you have while in male organizations, even gay men. Anywhere you go take a look around, and look for any places out are, and then check how they actually function? Windows, entrances, fire escapes, and so on.

Mindfulness. Let's talk about your community for a few minutes. Take note of the places you're walking through the city with your female friends. Get off messaging or off the phone if you're walking in a secluded or lush zone. Look around the surroundings, and mark any places where someone may hide. Be mindful of the entrances with a shrouding or a tree or trees, beneath an edifice, next to a private staircase that runs through the forest areas, or behind some supports or even trees. Be cautious in the event that you need to go through the left-hand side of the park. Make sure to walk in groups. Be aware of high-traffic areas, as well as parts of town that are beneficial to cars stopping to direct access to expressways or freeways. Look out for routes that traversing across isolated areas, fields, or old industrial sites. These regions offer OPPORTUNITY for sexual predators if they is forced to throw you into his vehicle or truck. Do not go there alone in the event that you are able to keep a safe distance from the area and avoid walking through it in the evening.

What are you carrying in your bag or in your pocket that could make a great weapon? Here are a few examples:

Your Keys. Place the key between two fingers, with the sharp end raised. Use it to strike or cut through the crotch region or eye zone. Keep your grip with the aim of making sure you don't lose it.

Hair Spray. Spray directly into the eyes and, if he's fast blinded, you can kick him or kick him as forcefully as you can into the crotch. Catch up by clenching your hand directly in the nose of his. Do not throw a punch from behind or take an attack.

Make sure you punch straight from your chest or your body, as the opponent may be able to see the punch coming in the event you try a swinging punch. Then strike it squarely. If the person is knocked down, do not wander around in a random manner, and be aware of where you're running. Be careful not to run to avoid a deadlock, or into a trap.

Be careful not to be snared on the back of a road. There is a chance that he's not far from others and you should be aware of the possibility of a label cooperation effort with a second or third attacker.

Pepper Spray. If you've got pepper spray, apply it to his eyes. Then, perform the same thing and kick or punch him in the crotch or step onto the instep (most amazing point-over-foot) using your rear.

Sharp Metal Nail File. Put it in his crotch, or try to cut him in the eye. Make use of your other hand to punch his crotch or grab his balls. In the event that the other hand is taken away by him use your knee to get into the crotch area and follow your foot and step. If it doesn't work, put your feet rear to the knee's at the top. Keep focusing on one as you could be causing harm or discomfort there. However you can hit anyone you are able to get to.

Head Butt. I would not recommend this in a tense situation. If you're holding both hands and you are unable to touch him with your feet, use the part of your forehead which forms your hairline. Draw your hair in reverse and then pummel the part of your head straight into his nose or even into his button. Bend your arms and deliver toward your body. Following you throw your the hands with clenched fingers (like mallets) into his nose. followed by a quick swing of both arms while clenching hands up and towards the sides of your hips or chest and then pummel the two hands of clench into his the crotch of his.

Conclusion

I would like to thank you for taking the time to read this book. At this point , I'd recommend you look for an academy of martial arts that can teach you proper grappling and striking. It is possible to inquire about whether they incorporate these pressure points as part of their classes. Particularly, I suggest finding schools that integrate the concepts of Kyusho Jitsu , such as Kyusho Kempo schools or Krav Maga.

If you're determined to do it, you must get training at a kempo academy which has Kyusho principles within the program. If you're in it for self-defense, then the krav maga or any self-defense training program that incorporates kyusho concepts will suffice.

This information here is only a basic guideline and won't make you extremely proficient. It is best to do them with an instructor to a certain extent, but not to a level of proficiency. You'll need the guidance by a real master to reach this level of proficiency.